Treat Your Own Tennis Elbow

by
Jim Johnson, PT

This book was designed to provide accurate information in regard to the subject matter covered. It is sold with the understanding that the author is not engaged in rendering medical, psychological, or other professional services. If expert assistance is required, the services of a professional should be sought.

Photographs by Christa Johnson
Drawings and Cover Art by Eunice Johnson

This edition published by
Dog Ear Publishing
4010 W. 86th Street, Ste H
Indianapolis, IN 46268

www.dogearpublishing.net

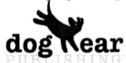

ISBN: 978-160844-390-1
Library of Congress Control Number:
This book is printed on acid-free paper.

Printed in the United States of America

How This Book Is Set Up

✓ Find out exactly what the problem is and where it's at in *Chapter 1*.

✓ Recognize what causes tennis elbow in *Chapter 2*.

✓ Be aware of the typical course that tennis elbow takes in *Chapter 3*.

✓ Learn how you can treat tennis elbow yourself in *Chapters 4 and 5*.

✓ Monitor your progress with the tools in *Chapter 6*.

Why Is The Print In This Book So Big?

People who read my books sometimes wonder why the print is so big in many of them. Some tend to think it's because I'm trying to make a little book bigger or a short book longer.

Actually, the main reason I use bigger print is for the same reason I intentionally write short books, usually under 100 pages–it's just plain easier to read and get the information quicker!

You see, the books I write address common, everyday problems that people of *all* ages have. In other words, the "typical" reader of my books could be a teenager, a busy housewife, a CEO, a construction worker, or a retired senior citizen with poor eyesight. Therefore, by writing books with larger print that are short and to the point, *everyone* can get the information quickly and with ease. After all, what good is a book full of useful information if nobody ever finishes it?

Table of Contents

While a lot of cases of tennis elbow do resolve in a short period of time, there are many that don't.

No doubt there is more than one reason why one person gets better and another worse, but being a busy clinician and researcher for over eighteen years, my guess is that a major factor is *whether you understand what's going on in your elbow or not.*

Why do I say this? Simply because the dysfunctional process that takes place in tennis elbow is not a complicated one. And once understood, interrupting this painful cycle is straightforward–giving the symptoms little reason to hang around .

This, then, is what **Treat Your Own Tennis Elbow** is all about. In the pages that follow, I will explain to you in simple terms, what's going on in your elbow *and* what you can do about it all on your own.

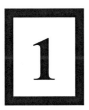 *This* is the Spot Where All the Trouble Is

Just for fun one time, I did a search to find out when the term "tennis elbow" first appeared in the medical literature. After a bit of tedious hunting, I narrowed my search down to an 1883 letter published in the British Medical Journal (Morris 1883). Interestingly, this painful condition was not exactly called "tennis elbow" at first, but rather coined "lawn tennis elbow."

However unlike the name, which has remained basically the same over the last hundred years and counting, our understanding of tennis elbow *has* changed a bit. Perhaps the first big breakthrough came in a 1979 journal article that finally pinpointed the exact location of tennis elbow…

How We Know Where the Problem Really Is

People with tennis elbow are all too familiar with that pain on the outside of their elbow. Problem is, there's *a lot* of things that make up the side of your elbow. For example, there's skin, nerves, many small muscles, some ligaments, and of course the bones. So how is it one can know for sure which structure, or structures, are causing all the pain?

Well, a good thought is to take a close look at some of the elbow's structures in people with tennis elbow, and check to see if there's anything out of the ordinary going on. While many surgeons have done this over the years, it really wasn't until the late 70's that an orthopedic surgeon by the name of Robert Nirschl ultimately got to the bottom of things.

According to his 1979 study, published in *The Journal of Bone and Joint Surgery*, Dr. Nirschl and his colleagues reported that after operating on eighty-two patients with tennis elbow, they noted one consistent finding: abnormalities in one of the small forearm muscles know as the *extensor carpi radialis brevis*.

At this point, some readers may be wondering just how Dr. Nirschl and his colleagues managed to discover the problem muscle when no one else could? Well, apparently other surgeons in the past didn't typically lift up the extensor carpi radialis *longus* muscle while operating on tennis elbow patients, which one must do in order to see the abnormal part of the extensor carpi radialis *brevis* muscle underneath. Therefore, if you don't lift up the longus, you can't see the whole brevis. Over time, other researchers have confirmed Dr. Nirschl's findings using a wide variety of methods such as ultrasound (De Zordo 2009), MRI scans (Potter 1995), and of course more surgical observations (Regan 1992).

The Little Muscle That Causes *Big* Problems

I know, at this point you're saying to yourself, "Extensor carpi what?" Clearly a little explaining is in order. First things first. Where is it and what does it look like? The following basic picture should answer both of these questions:

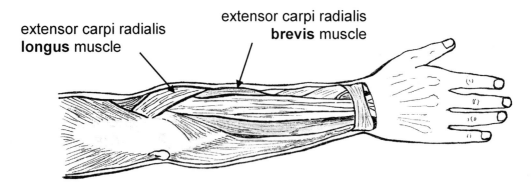

extensor carpi radialis
longus muscle

extensor carpi radialis
brevis muscle

Figure 1. Looking at outer part of the extensor carpi radialis
brevis on the *right* arm.

So what do think of that extensor carpi radialis brevis? There are a few things I want you to pick up from the picture. Number one is, while I have intentionally avoided a highly detailed picture in order to keep things simple, you can easily get the idea that you have many small muscles that make up your forearm *and* that the extensor carpi radialis brevis is near the top. Secondly, you can also see that it runs lengthwise up and down your forearm and seems to "dive" in under the longus muscle. But where is it going?

To make a long story short, the extensor carpi radialis brevis is headed to one of your arm bones. This is because muscles are like rubber bands and must be firmly attached at both of their ends in order to contract and work. Therefore, to tell you *exactly* where the extensor carpi radialis brevis attaches to, means that you're first going to have to know a little bit about your arm bones. Here are a couple of pictures to give you an idea of what bones are in your arm:

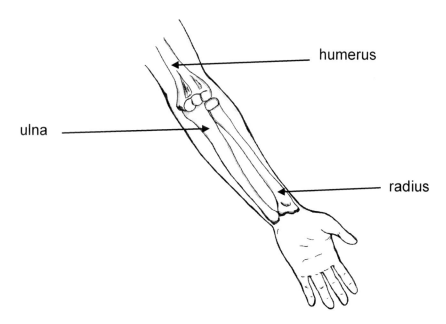

Figure 2. The bones that make up your *left* arm.

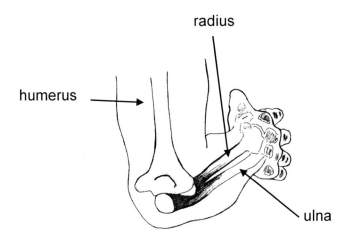

Figure 3. A rear view of how your *right* arm bones fit together.

As you can see, your arm is made up of three bones, one upper arm bone (the *humerus*), and two forearm bones (the *ulna*, and the *radius*). You don't need to memorize these little guy's names, just get a general sense of their location in your arm.

Okay, now that you're a little more familiar with the arm bones, next up is, which one does the extensor carpi radialis brevis attach to? Well, it's the one called your *humerus*, or upper arm bone. The following picture shows you pretty accurately where the extensor carpi radialis brevis attaches to on this peculiar looking bone:

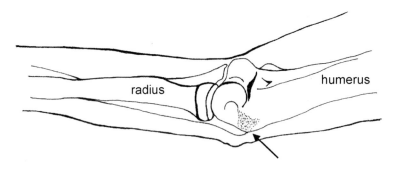

Figure 4. Arrow points to the dotted area on the outer elbow
where the extensor carpi radialis brevis attaches to.
Note that the picture is of a *left* arm.

Wow, we sure have covered a lot of ground so far! In case all of this is a bit overwhelming, let's quickly review a few things to make sure we're all on the same page.

The problem in tennis elbow is with a little forearm muscle called your *extensor carpi radialis brevis.* We know this because it's the muscle where surgeons see all kinds of abnormalities. One of its ends attaches to your upper arm bone called the *humerus.* Know too that muscles have *tendons* that help them stay connected to the bones, which is a tough white tissue that goes *between* the muscle and the bone, thus keeping it firmly attached.

Figure 5 shows us exactly how the tendon connects your extensor carpi radialis brevis to your upper arm bone. *It is this tendon part where all the abnormalities are found in people with tennis elbow.*

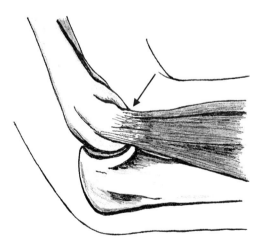

Figure 5. Arrow points to the tendon that connects the extensor carpi radialis brevis to the upper arm bone. This is the spot where abnormalities are found in people with tennis elbow.

What Your Extensor Carpi Radialis Brevis Does

By this time, most readers are probably wondering what the heck this muscle does. I mean if it can cause this much trouble, it must do something *really* important, right?

Absolutely. The extensor carpi radialis brevis does have an important job. In fact, it has several. The first big one is that it is involved in *extension* of your wrist. What's wrist extension? Check out these photos…

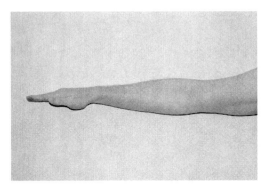

Here's your wrist in a *neutral* or middle position.
As you can see, it's straight as an arrow.

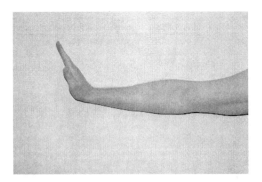

Now here's your wrist in *extension*, or in a "pulled up" position.
As you can see, it's bending upwards towards your head.

Yes, it's true! The extensor carpi radialis brevis works very hard *every* time you move your wrist into extension (which is up towards your head as in the last picture). Because it does this, it's called a *wrist extensor* in medical lingo.

So is that all it does? Well, not quite, it's also really active every time you open and close your hand, *and* especially when you do this…

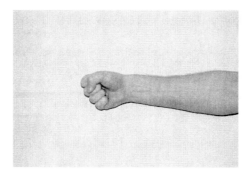

That's right, another big job of your extensor carpi radialis brevis is to help you *grip* things.

So how do we know all this to be true, that the extensor carpi radialis brevis works hard to open and close your hand, grip things, and pulls your wrist up? Mostly from researchers doing *electromyographic* or *EMG studies*. By inserting needles directly into the extensor carpi radialis brevis of a subject, and then asking them to move their wrist and hand around, the electrical activity of the muscle can be measured to identify the motions which it is most active in.

Of note, most of the EMG studies done on the extensor carpi radialis brevis were conducted some time ago (for example Radonjic 1971 and McFarland 1962). EMG's are pretty straighforward tests, and once you've shown consistently that a muscle does something, there's not much point in duplicating the results too many more times!

Key Points

✓ the main problem in tennis elbow is with a forearm muscle known as the extensor carpi radialis brevis

✓ the tendon of the extensor carpi radialis brevis, where it attaches to your upper arm bone, is where all the abnormalities are seen in people with tennis elbow

✓ the extensor carpi radialis brevis muscle is especially working hard when you open and close your hand, grip things, and pull up your wrist

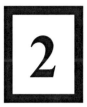

What Went Wrong
At Your Elbow

Many readers, in search of relief, have probably run across the term "lateral epicondylitis" at one time or another.   For those not in the know, *lateral epicondylitis* is the medical term for tennis elbow. But how did they come up with a name like that for tennis elbow?

Well, the word "lateral" in medical terminology is used to describe things that are out to the side. "Epicondylitis", on the other hand, can actually be broken down into two parts. The first part, "epicondyl" is short for *epicondyle*, which refers to the bony "bumps" that are on the inside and outside of your upper arm bone. Figure 6 shows you your medial (inside) and lateral (outside) epicondyles, which are basically just two bony "bumps" that the muscles attach themselves to:

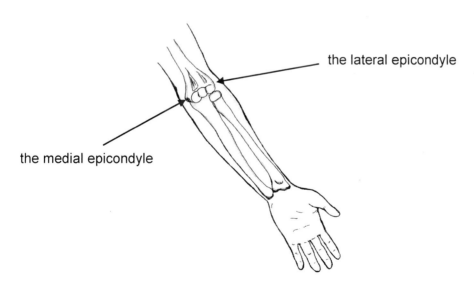

the lateral epicondyle

the medial epicondyle

Figure 6. Arrows point to your medial and lateral epicondyles of your *left* arm.

So now that you know what the first half of the word "epicondylitis" means, what about the second half, "itis"? To put it simply, it's just a word that is commonly tacked on to the end of *another* word and means inflammation.

Therefore, if you put it *all* together, lateral epicondylitis literally means inflammation of the outer condyle–which is the general area where your extensor carpi radialis brevis attaches itself to. And since we're talking about various names for tennis elbow, the other most commonly used one you'll hear is "elbow tendonitis"–meaning inflammation of a tendon at the elbow.

Now while these terms *appear* to make sense, I have a bone to pick with both of them. The problem? *They're both inaccurate*. Why you say? Simply because both of them use the word "itis" which implies that tennis elbow is an inflammatory condition–*but it's not!*

Surprised? You're not alone. Confused? You won't be for long. Skeptical? Well, I consider that a good thing. Let me explain why tennis elbow has nothing to do with you having an *inflamed* tendon...

What the Microscope Tells Us About Tennis Elbow

Approaching this matter scientifically, as we do everything in this book, to say that something is "inflammed" means that we should be able to find some hard evidence of inflammation. Without getting too caught up in details, inflammation can be broken down into two general patterns, *acute* and *chronic*. Here's the difference between the two:

- *acute inflammation* is an immediate and early response to tissue injury. It comes on quick, but lasts for minutes, hours, or a few days. Neutrophils are the major kind of cells that are involved in acute inflammation.

- *chronic inflammation* is inflammation of a prolonged duration, such as weeks or months. Some of the major types of cells that are involved in chronic inflammation include macrophages, lymphocytes, and plasma cells.

Now it's *not* important to know all about the different types of cells, although you may be interested to know that a lot of them are simply different types of white blood cells. What is important, however, is to know that these are exactly the kinds of cells we should be able to find in people with tennis elbow *if* the tendon or muscle is indeed "inflammed"–since these are the cells directly involved in the body's inflammatory process. With this knowledge now in hand, let's look at the results of a few studies from the published literature where researchers have closely examined the extensor carpi radialis brevis in people with tennis elbow...

study	*# of samples*	*average duration of symptoms*	*major histological findings reported*
Potter 1995	**20**	**18 months**	**-disorganization and /or disruption of collagen fibers, mucoid degeneration, neovascularization** **-no evidence of acute or chronic inflammation**
Verhaar 1993	**63**	**avg. of 50 weeks of non-operative treatment**	**-vascular proliferation, mucoid degeneration** **-no evidence of any inflammatory reaction**
Regan 1992	**11**	**26 months**	**-vascular proliferation, hyaline degeneration, fibroblastic proliferation, calcific debris** **-no evidence of inflammatory cells**
Nirschl 1979	**88**	**36 months**	**-immature fibroblastic and vascular infiltration**

Well, as you can see from the table, it doesn't look like researchers have reported finding many of the cells that are directly involved in the inflammatory process. Therefore, without some cellular proof of an inflammatory response, one has *no basis* to accurately say that there is indeed "inflammation" when one has tennis elbow. The evidence just isn't there!

> ***Critical point:*** Inflammation does *not* appear to be a major feature of tennis elbow, especially in patients that have been suffering with this condition for many months.

On the other hand, what researches *have found* when taking a piece of tendon at surgery and looking at it later under a microscope, are signs of **failed tendon healing**. Glancing back at the table, you'll see that researchers noted, among other things...

- *disrupted and disorganized collagen fibers.* Collagen is a main ingredient that makes up your connective tissues–and it's having a hard time coming together properly in the tendon!

- *fibroblastic proliferation.* Fibroblast cells work like a "construction crew" to make connective tissue. We see a lot of these little guys, some abnormal, floating around in the tendons of tennis elbow sufferers–so they're obviously looking for work!

- *vascular proliferation.* Lots of blood vessels, many of which are abnormal and immature, are found in the area–a sign that tendon healing is trying to take place!

But enough written descriptions. Let's take a look at a few drawings to get a better "picture" of what's going on...

Here is what a normal tendon looks like up close…

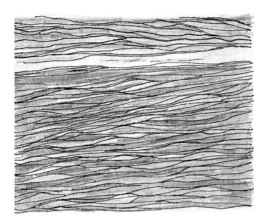

Notice how straight and organized the tendon fibers are. That's the way things are *suppose* to be. Now check out this drawing…

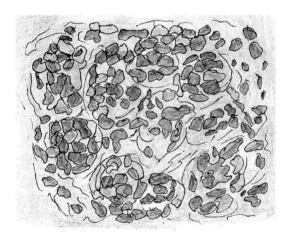

Wow! So that's what your tendon looks like when you have tennis elbow. Looks a little different from the first one, doesn't it? What a mess! As you can tell, there's *a lot* of disorganization going on there. Your body is trying to repair itself, but can't quite get its act together. But how did the tendon become so abnormal?

How Tendons Get Messed Up

The answer to the question, "How did the tendon become so abnormal?" can be answered in one word: *overuse*. The story goes something like this.

First, know that as you use your arms throughout the day, you're contracting the muscles, which are in turn pulling hard on your tendons (remember that tendons help connect the muscles to the bones). And, just like most things in your body, the tendons and muscles need time (at some point) to rest and repair themselves from this normal daily wear and tear.

Therefore, if you work your tendons and muscles, and give them *enough* time to recover each day, they're going to stay in good shape. We could then say that your muscles and tendons are "keeping up" with your activities. And all is well.

Now let's say you have a day where you've worked your tendons and muscles *more* than normal, or you're just using them in a way they're simply not used to. For example, maybe you did a lot more typing that day, or maybe you just tried a new sport after work like racquetball. Well, of course this is going to cause *more* wear and tear than the muscles and tendons are normally used to, right?

Well, here's where the problems can start. **If** you give your arm muscles and tendons time to rest and recover (meaning that they have time to make the necessary repairs from this increased stress) *before* using them a lot again, your tendons will be able to "keep up", stay in good working order, and will continue looking like this:

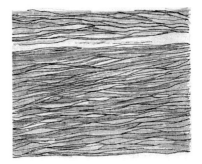

On the other hand, let's say you *continue* to repeatedly work your muscles and tendons harder than usual and they don't get enough time off to recover and make repairs. What will happen to them then? Well, *over time* your tendons will be unable to "keep up" with the activities you ask them to do, start to become internally disorganized, and will eventually end up looking like this:

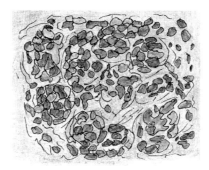

The moral of the story? The main problem in tennis elbow is one of **failed tendon healing**. And the tendon has failed to heal because it was repeatedly put through stressful activities–and then not given enough repair time.

Avoid Doing Too Much of These Activities

So the next question some readers might have is, "Are there any kinds of activities that can cause tennis elbow?"

Well, first of all, keep in mind that it's not really the activity in and of itself that's the real problem, but rather the fact that someone does *too much* of it. It's kind of like walking on your heels. Walk on your heels for a few feet and you're fine. Walk around all day on your heels…

Having said that, there are some motions of the wrist that *do* work the extensor carpi radialis brevis tendon more than others. Therefore, doing too many activities that involve such motions *could* make you more prone to getting tennis elbow.

And what are these motions? Well, remember from Chapter One that the extensor carpi radialis brevis is highly active when you *open and close your hand*, *grip things*, and *pull up your wrist*. So, here are some common activities which involve these motions…

- racquet sports such as racquetball or tennis
- typing
- carpentry work
- using a screwdriver
- repetitive lifting
- computer work
- frequent handshaking
- gardening

These are just a few examples. Note that you can get tennis elbow, not only from playing tennis, but also from other repetitive activities such as using a screwdriver excessively. I guess then you *could* call it "screwdriver elbow"…

Seriously though, the key point here is to remember that *any* activity which involves you frequently opening and closing your hand, continuously gripping things, or constantly pulling up your wrist repeatedly *is* working that elbow tendon to varying degrees–and thus puts a person at risk for getting tennis elbow.

Key Points

✓ inflammation does *not* appear to be a major feature of tennis elbow, especially in patients that have been suffering with this condition for many months

✓ we know this because if researchers take a piece of tendon from people suffering from tennis elbow, and look at it closely under a microscope, they can't find any signs of inflammation

✓ instead, the main problem in tennis elbow is one of *failed tendon healing*

✓ the tendon has failed to heal because it was repeatedly put through stressful activities–and then not given enough repair time

✓ activities where you are frequently opening and closing your hand, continuously gripping things, or constantly pulling your wrist up repeatedly, stresses the tendon and can put you at risk fact for getting tennis elbow

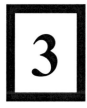

What Your Prognosis Is

Prognosis can be defined as a prediction of the probable course and outcome of a disease. Practically speaking, it's your chances of recovery. So if you have tennis elbow, what are your chances of getting back to normal?

Scientifically speaking, the only way to know for sure how long tennis elbow typically lasts, is to conduct what is called a *natural history study*. Natural history studies attempt to find out exactly how long a disease (or problem) will last on its own, naturally, without interference, by following a group of patients over time that receive *no medical treatment*. Problem is, while there are natural history studies for many different medical conditions, none have been done on tennis elbow. Apparently tennis elbow sufferers are hesitant to skip medical treatment for the sake of science!

But before you get too discouraged, let me tell you what you *will* find when sifting through the research–studies on how people with tennis elbow do over the long run *when managed non-operatively* (without surgery). The studies go something like this:

- researchers record how bad a group of patient's symptoms are
- next, patients get some kind of treatment
- patients are followed for a period of time, and their symptoms are re-checked to see how long it took them to get better

While you won't be able to figure out the *true* natural course of tennis elbow from these kinds of studies, you will be able to get enough information to tell someone about how long their tennis elbow might last after they start treatment for it. Let's have a quick look at some of the best studies done in this area that have fairly long follow-up periods…

What Will Happen If You
Take the "Wait and See" Approach

Some of the best kind of research you can look at to determine how long tennis elbow lasts is what I call the "wait and see" studies. I call them this because in these studies, patients are randomly divided up into several groups, one of which is called a "wait and see" group.

If you're in this particular group, you get little or no treatment, which means you're basically just keeping an eye on your tennis elbow so you can "wait and see" what it's going to do. Here are a couple of examples:

Study #1

- 198 patients with tennis elbow were randomly sent to one of three groups for 6-weeks of treatment (Bisset 2006)

- one group got physical therapy which consisted of manipulation and exercise

- another group got up to two steroid injections

- the "wait and see" group just got advice on how to manage their tennis elbow at the start of the study

- patients were checked on in one year to see how they were doing

- the physical therapy group had a success rate of 94% , the group that got steroid injections had a success rate of 68%, and the "wait and see" group had a success rate of 90%

I'm sure the first thing that caught your eye was the fact that 90% of the people in the "wait and see" group were better in one year's time, when just given basic advice on how to manage their tennis elbow. Sound too good to be true? Well it is. Further examination of the study results reveals that over this one year follow-up period, 55% of those in the "wait and see" group sought out *additional* treatments for their tennis elbow, which consisted of conservative, non-surgical treatments such as elbow braces or acupuncture.

Hmm. Let's take a look at another "wait and see" study to see what they found…

Study #2

- 185 patients with tennis elbow were randomly sent to one of three groups for 6-weeks of treatment (Smidt 2002)

- one group got physical therapy which consisted of ultrasound, friction massage, and exercise

- another group got up to three steroid injections

- the "wait and see group" got medications and advice on how to manage their tennis elbow at the start of the study

- patients were checked on in one year to see how they were doing

- the physical therapy group had a success rate of 91%, the group that got steroid injections had a success rate of 69%, and the "wait and see" group had a success rate of 83%

Looks like in this study, 83% of subjects in the "wait and see" group, who got just advice and medication, got better within a year's time. But here again, we have to wonder, how many of them went out and sought *other* treatments over that one year period? Any guesses?

24%. Which of course means that simply giving advice and medications to treat tennis elbow simply wasn't good enough to take care of the pain in 24% of people in the "wait and see" group–and so they went out and got additional treatments, like an elbow support.

So what are we to make of all these results and numbers? Anything useful amongst the statistics for the tennis elbow sufferer? Well, several conclusions *can* be drawn:

- the majority of people with tennis elbow can and do get better within a year *with conservative, non-surgical treatments*

- in a significant amount of tennis elbow sufferers, it takes more than just medications and basic medical advice to get better

So the million dollar question is, if the majority of tennis elbow sufferers can get better with treatment by the one-year mark, which treatments work best?

Well, the studies we've just gone over don't really give us many specific answers in that department–however there are studies that do. And that's exactly what the remainder of this book is all about: the best treatments to get rid of tennis elbow in the shortest amount of time–*that you can do on your own.*

 # A Surefire Way to Help Your Elbow Finally Heal

Probably the single most important piece of information to know when it comes to unlocking the mystery of getting rid of tennis elbow, is realizing that the main problem is actually one of *failed tendon healing*. Therefore, it logically follows, that a successful treatment must be one that creates a healing environment for the extensor carpi radialis brevis tendon to finally repair itself. But what exactly can you do to create this healing environment?

How to *Eliminate* the Harmful Stress on Your Tendon

This first approach is a no-brainer–but one I can't neglect to mention. Figure out what activities you're doing that are stressing and aggravating your elbow tendon *and stop doing them*.

While simple enough, doing this one thing alone is a giant step towards full recovery. With tennis elbow being caused by overuse, simply stopping the irritating activity immediately takes the stress off the extensor carpi radialis brevis tendon–*and gives it a chance to begin the healing process.*

Of course most readers won't need a lot of advice to figure out which activities to stop doing–that's because the ones that cause the most problems are the ones that hurt the most! The short story goes like this: if it hurts, don't do it.

On the other hand, the long story goes like this. Recall from previous chapters, that the extensor carpi radialis brevis muscle is working hard and pulling on your healing tendon, *especially when you're opening and closing your hand, gripping things, and pulling up your wrist*. Therefore, since these motions are the worst offenders, pinpoint which activities you're doing that involve them–and skip them altogether.

How to *Decrease* the Harmful Stress on Your Tendon

While eliminating the harmful stresses is obvious and guaranteed to get your tendon headed in the right direction, there is one problem: it's much easier said than done. That's because, for a lot of people, the aggravating motions that are causing the problem are an essential part of their day.

Perhaps someone has a child they have to pick up a lot, or maybe a person does a lot of gripping and twisting at work which is vital to getting their job done. In many cases, it can be *really* hard to stop using your arm the way you're used to using it every day. So what then? Is all lost?

Not quite. If you can't *eliminate* the stress on your extensor carpi radialis brevis tendon, then the next best thing is to *decrease* the stress. How? Easy. By using a *brace*. Here's a picture of what could be your tendon's best friend:

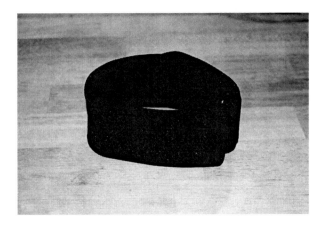

As you can see, the brace is basically a piece of soft material that is made to wrap around your forearm. I'll be going over in more detail later exactly how to put one on, but for now, just know that you place it around your forearm and it's held snugly in place by velcro.

While it may not look like much, this little brace has been proven to help tennis elbow sufferers *a lot*. But what exactly do I mean when I say "proven"?

Well, in medicine, if you want to prove that a drug or any other kind of treatment really works, the best way to test it out is in *a randomized controlled trial*. This research method produces the highest form of proof showing whether or not a treatment is truly effective–and that the results are not simply due to some other factor (s). Let me give you a basic example of one.

Say you want to prove that taking Vitamin C gets rid of tennis elbow. Well, first you would go out and find, say, 100 people with tennis elbow, and then *randomize* them into two groups of fifty–which means you pick them at random to go into one group or the other. Doing it this way keeps things fair because it makes sure that each subject has an equal chance of being put into either group–and that no one was purposely put here or there where they might do better or worse.

Next, you make one group the treatment group (meaning that they get to take the Vitamin C) and the other one a control group (meaning that they get either a comparison treatment, or better yet, *no* treatment at all). Take note that the control group is one of the most important parts of the randomized controlled trial because it allows you to compare how people do when they *don't* get the treatment you're testing out.

Okay, so now you're ready to start your own randomized controlled trial to test out the theory that taking Vitamin C does indeed get rid of tennis elbow. You let the people in the treatment group take their Vitamin C, let the people in the control group go about their normal business, and then check on everybody in, say, six weeks to see how they are doing.

If, at the end of the six-week trial, the Vitamin C group has significantly less arm pain than the control group, you can now say with confidence that taking Vitamin C is indeed an effective treatment for tennis elbow. That's because everyone at the start of the study had the same condition (tennis elbow), an equal chance of getting into either group, and the group that took the Vitamin C were the only ones who got better. Therefore, we assume it must have been that Vitamin C!

On the other hand, if the group that took the Vitamin C and the control group both ended up with the *same* level of arm pain at the end of the six-week study, then we would have to say that taking Vitamin C *does not* work at all. This is simply because both groups ended up with the same amount of arm pain whether they took Vitamin C or not. Pretty nifty set-up, huh?

At this point, some readers might be wondering just why I'm dragging them through all this research mumbo-jumbo. Well, it's not because I'm trying to turn you into junior scientists. No, it's for two *very* important reasons.

The first one is so you will have every confidence that the recommended treatments in **Treat Your Own Tennis Elbow** really *do* work. Now that you know what a randomized controlled trial is, and that it produces the highest form of proof in medicine that a treatment is really effective, it will mean much more to you when I say that the conservative treatments contained in this book have been shown in randomized controlled trials to effectively decrease the symptoms of tennis elbow. Unfortunately, I doubt you'll find many other self-help books that are based on this kind of evidence.

The second reason? Well, I guess the teacher in me likes to educate people about the randomized controlled trial so that they will become more informed consumers. If you're like me, you work at least forty hours a week and quite possibly have a family to take care of. We all work hard for our money and I think it's really unfair when someone asks us to spend some of it on a product or service that makes miraculous claims without a shred of real evidence!

However now that *you* know exactly what to look for when deciding on a treatment for a particular problem (one or more randomized controlled trials that show effectiveness), you'll be able to tell if it's something you want to invest your time and money in, or if it's clearly a hit or miss venture. Okay, back to the brace…

So what do the randomized controlled trials have to say about these things? Well, let's have a brief look at a couple of studies…

Study #1

- 61 patients with tennis elbow were randomly assigned to one of three groups (Haker 1993)

- one group got up to 2 steroid injections

- another group wore a rigid splint for three months which immobilized the wrist

- the last group wore a brace for three months

- no other treatments or drugs were used throughout the trial

- patients were checked on in three months to see how they were doing

- 50% of subjects who wore the brace had a good or excellent outcome, compared to 21% in the splint group and 63% in the steroid injection group

---

It appears from this study, that *half* the people, who did nothing more than just put a simple little brace on each day, found relief from their tennis elbow in a matter of weeks. I'd say that at least makes the brace worth a good look as a low-cost, conservative, do-it-yourself option. Let's see what some other studies have found…

Study #2

- 180 patients with tennis elbow were randomly assigned to one of three groups for 6-weeks of treatment (Struijs 2004)

- one group got physical therapy which consisted of ultrasound, friction massage, and exercises

- another group wore a brace

- the last group got physical therapy *and* wore a brace

- patients were checked on in 6-weeks to see how they were doing

- the physical therapy group had a success rate of 50%, the group that wore the brace had a success rate of 40%, and the group that got both the physical therapy plus the brace had a success rate of 45%

Here again, it looks like around half the people who tried the brace got good relief in a matter of weeks. Also of interest, is the fact that the people who simply wore a brace did almost as well as those subjects who had a more sophisticated (and expensive) treatment.

Okay. Say you want to try out one of these little gizmos. Where do you get one and how do you go about using it? Well, first know that if you're looking in a store or on the internet for one, they do go by various names. Probably some of the most common ones you'll see are "counterforce brace", "elbow brace", "elbow support", "elbow band", or "elbow strap". Regardless of the name, however, *they all work the same way and they all do the same thing.*

Key Points

✓ there are no true natural history studies to tell us what will happens to tennis elbow over the long run when it goes untreated

✓ "wait and see" studies tell us that the prognosis of tennis elbow is good, with some 80% to 90% of people getting better in a year's time *with* treatment

✓ "wait and see" studies also reveal that for a significant amount of tennis elbow sufferers, it takes more than just medications and basic medical advice to get better

When choosing one, also be aware that *I know of no research showing one particular brand to be better than another.* My advice is to pick one that fits your price range and is comfortable. If you're getting one in a store, such as a drug store (pharmacy), or retail store (look in the sporting goods section), more often than not you can try one on before buying to get a general idea of how it feels.

More importantly than the brand, however, is *how* you wear the brace. To make a long story short, placement is *everything* if you want to get the best results. Just so there's no confusion, here's a picture of my arm with the brace applied correctly:

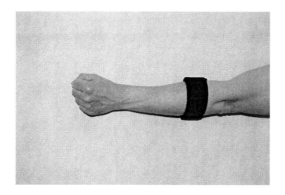

Note that the brace is worn high up near the elbow, which is over the area where the extensor carpi radialis brevis muscle is. As you might have guessed, the idea is to put the brace snugly over this muscle. Here's our Mr. Arm again to give you an "X-ray" look at where the brace goes:

extensor carpi radialis brevis muscle

brace placed over extensor carpi radialis brevis muscle

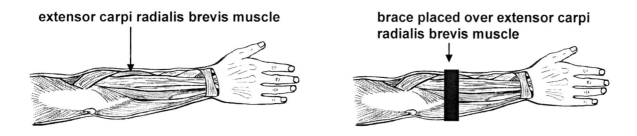

At this point, some readers may be worried that they won't get the brace *exactly* over the extensor carpi radialis brevis muscle. Not to worry. Because these braces are fairly wide, you'll hit the target as long you place it like the picture. However note what will *not* work…

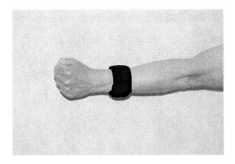

Too low! You can use it as a bracelet *after* you've recovered…

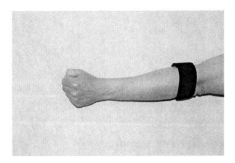

Too high! Gets in the way of elbow bending…

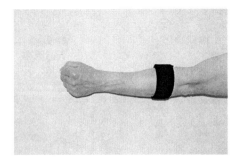

Ahh, just right.

Now that you know how to place the brace correctly on your arm, how tight should it be? Well, probably the best way to describe how tight is to say that the band should be snug, but not so tight that it cuts off the circulation or becomes uncomfortable. When applied properly, the brace should stay put and *not* slide up or down on your arm either.

Although there is unfortunately no research to tell us for sure how this handy little brace works, one popular theory is that the tension of the band over the extensor carpi radialis brevis muscle reduces how hard it's able to pull on the injured tendon. And so, the less the muscle is able to pull on the tendon, the less force there is being applied to the tendon–giving it more of a chance to rest and repair itself. That's why I recommend you wear the brace during the day, whenever you're going to be doing activities that might stress your elbow.

Perhaps the best thing about using the brace is that as soon as you put it on, it goes to work for you *right away*. We know this because studies have found…

- people with tennis elbow immediately have less pain with wrist bending after putting the brace on (Ng 2004)

- people with tennis elbow actually have increased wrist strength and can suddenly grip things tighter after putting the brace on (Wadsworth 1989)

- people with tennis elbow who put on a brace instantly showed an increase in pain-free grip strength (Burton 1985)

While wearing the brace will help your symptoms and allow your elbow to heal, don't let it trick you into thinking you're Superman either. Controlling the *duration* and *intensity* of aggravating activities that you do is also crucial. What do I mean by this? Consider the following example…

- say you have to move 20 boxes around

- instead of lifting 20 boxes in one hour, you could try controlling the *intensity* of this activity by lifting only 10 boxes in one hour. Because you lifted fewer boxes per an hour, you have decreased the stress on your elbow tendon.

- instead of lifting all 20 boxes in one day, you could try controlling the *duration* of this activity by lifting 10 boxes one day, and then 10 the next. Because you lifted fewer boxes in a day, you have decreased the stress on your elbow tendon.

This tactic works so well because it is the exact *opposite* process of what caused your tennis elbow in the first place. As you recall, tennis elbow is an overuse injury where the tendon was stressed more frequently and/or more intensely over a given amount of time than it could recover from–resulting in a failed healing process (and lots of pain).

On the other hand, the above approach seeks to control the stresses placed on the tendon by pacing how long and how intense the tendon gets worked in a given amount of time. While the above scenario is a simple example, the same principles can be easily applied to everything from how many games of tennis you play in a day, to how much typing or hammering one does. Just something to keep in mind…

Key Points

- ✓ if possible, eliminate entirely those activities that involve repetitive opening and closing of your hand, gripping things, and pulling up your wrist

- ✓ use a brace to decrease the stress on your elbow tendon

- ✓ according to randomized controlled trials, about half of tennis elbow sufferers who wear a brace, and use no other treatment, will recover *within* a 6 to 12-week time frame

- ✓ the brace is applied over the extensor carpi radialis brevis muscle, and worn snugly during the day when performing activities stressful to the tendon

- ✓ controlling the duration and intensity of aggravating activities is also a good strategy to take stress off the extensor carpi radialis brevis tendon and help it heal

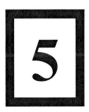

Doing *This* Will Repair The Damage

There are two basic strategies used in this book to help you recover from tennis elbow. The first one is to set up the right environment for the tendon to begin its healing process–which is done by eliminating (or lowering) the harmful stresses that are being placed on it. This we've just discussed in the last chapter.

When that is put into action, the tendon no longer has to use up all its resources recovering from harmful stresses. Instead, the extensor carpi radialis brevis tendon can now begin expending its energy on the repair process. And this brings us to the second strategy–*improving the quality of your tendon tissue.*

The Healing Changes That Need To Take Place

Improve the quality of the tendon tissue. Hmm. What exactly does that mean? Well, recall from Chapter 2…

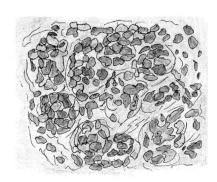

This is what your extensor carpi radialis brevis tendon looks like now.

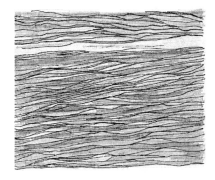

This is what your extensor carpi radialis brevis tendon needs to look like.

The goal is to get from the picture on the left to the picture on the right. But how? Well, by *reversing* the disorganized changes that have taken place. So what we need here is a treatment that can...

- encourage a new blood vessel supply

- promote the formation of healing tissue cells
  (such as fibroblasts) and healing materials (such as collagen)

- make the newly formed tissue line up properly

If we can somehow "jump start" things, and make these changes begin to happen, well, it'll be just a matter of time before your tennis elbow heals up *and* becomes a thing of the past. But is there one single treatment that can pull all of this off? Absolutely! It's called *exercise*...

It Works!

Some readers may find it hard to believe that exercise is the cure for an *overused* tendon. I admit this concept does seem a bit strange, but exercise has been proven to work in randomized controlled trials. Here's a good example:

- 39 patients with chronic tennis elbow were randomly sent to one of two groups for 6 to 8-weeks of treatment (Pienimaki 1996)

- one group got a home exercise program of stretching and strengthening exercises

- the other group got ultrasound two to three times a week

- no other treatments were allowed

- at the 8-week follow-up, patients in the exercise group had significantly less pain, less sleep disturbances, better grip strength, and were able to do more of their usual work

---

There are two very interesting things in particular about this randomized controlled trial. First, patients in this study got better when they did their exercises *at home*. This is extremely good news for many people, because it proves that long-term tennis elbow sufferers *can* get better by doing an exercise program on their own–which is what this book is all about!

The second thing to note is that this study tackled *chronic* (long-term) tennis elbow sufferers. In fact, many had pain for over an entire year. Not an easy bunch to get better, especially since many of them had *already* tried many other treatments such as immobilization, injections, medications, etc.–all with no success. Exercise, however, did succeed in doing the trick where others failed. But not all exercise programs are created equal…

The Ideal Exercise Program For Tennis Elbow

What are some good exercises for tennis elbow? Ask two physical therapists and I doubt you'll get two identical answers. Of course this doesn't necessarily mean that one therapist is right and the other one wrong–because there's always more than one way to skin a cat.

What I would argue, however, is that there are exercises programs for tennis elbow that are clearly more *ideal* than others. While there are many different kinds of exercises to choose from, it is my *opinion* that the best, conservative, do-it-yourself, exercise program should be:

- proven to actually work in one or more
  randomized controlled trials

and

- get the best results with the least amount
  of exercises

To that end, this book will recommend that you do two exercises for your tennis elbow, one *stretching* exercise and one *strengthening* exercise. Now the stretching exercise is just that—a simple static stretch for the extensor carpi radialis brevis muscle and tendon. However the strengthening exercise is a bit different. To do it, you won't be lifting a weight, but rather *lowering* it.

If this sounds funny to you, you're not alone. Despite its lack of popular use, this particular type of strengthening technique has been well studied and is called *eccentric* exercise. So what exactly is that?

Well, to make a long story short, when you lift a weight up, your muscle has *concentrically* contracted (and the fibers shorten), and when you lower the weight, the muscle *eccentrically* contracts (and the fibers lengthen).

Cutting edge research is now showing eccentric exercise to be very beneficial for people with "tendinitis" conditions, such as tennis elbow. Let's have a quick look at a few of these studies and then we'll be moving right to the exercises…

Study #1

- 94 subjects with chronic tennis elbow were randomly assigned to one of three groups for 6-weeks of treatment (Martinez-Silvestrini 2005). All exercises were done at home.

- one group did a stretching exercise

- another group did a strengthening exercise that involved just lifting the weight (the concentric part) without lowering it–plus a stretching exercise

- the last group did a strengthening exercise, that involved just lowering the weight (the eccentric part)–plus a stretching exercise

- all groups were allowed to use a brace, advised to avoid aggravating activities, and iced as needed

- patients were checked on in 6-weeks to see how they were doing

- 86% of subjects completed the study. All three groups improved significantly with no differences between the groups

There are lots of things to note in this study, but as far as analyzing the effects of eccentric exercise on chronic tennis elbow sufferers, this randomized controlled trial tells us that lowering a weight is just as effective as doing the raising part. Here's another interesting study…

Study #2

- 75 patients with tennis elbow were sequentially allocated to one of three groups for 4-weeks of treatment (Stasinopoulos 2006)

- one group was treated with friction massage and manipulation

- another group got light therapy

- the last group did eccentric exercises and static stretching

- patients were checked on in 4-weeks to see how they were doing

- there were no dropouts and those that did the eccentric exercise and static stretching showed the largest reductions in pain, as well as the greatest improvement in function

---

Note that this is a controlled study where researchers used *sequential allocation* to divide up its subjects. Instead of randomly assigning patients to groups, the first one that walked through the door that met the study criteria was assigned to group one, the second one that walked through the door was assigned to group two, and the third assigned to group three. When the fourth patient was available, the assignment started back to placing subjects into group one, and so on. While not true randomization, it's still pretty random–and yet *another* convincing study showing us that static stretching and eccentric exercise can hold their own.

Okay, we're almost done with laying the foundation of our exercise treatment. One last study to go…

Study #3

- 40 patients with tennis elbow were sequentially allocated to one of two groups for 4-weeks of treatment (Manias 2006)

- one group was treated with eccentric exercise and static stretching

- the other group was treated with eccentric exercise and static stretching–plus ice at the end of the treatment

- no other treatments were allowed during the study, including medications

- patients rated their pain on a scale of 0 to 10 where 0 was "least pain imaginable" and 10 was "worst pain imaginable

- patients were checked on in 4-weeks to see how they were doing

- both groups had less pain, dropping about 7 units on the scale from the start of the study

---

This controlled study is a good one to know about because it shows us that it's a waste of our time to add icing to a program of eccentric exercise and stretching. Of course you learned in Chapter 2 that there's no inflammation involved in tennis elbow–so you probably saw that one coming...

Another thing I need to add is, like the last study, there were no dropouts, which means that none of the 40 patients got fed up and quit. Instead, everyone completed the study and dropped about 7 units on the pain scale. That means that if a patient came in with a pain score of "10" (worst pain imaginable), they walked away a "3" within 4-week's time. Not bad. The low dropout rates we're seeing in these studies are a good indication that eccentric exercise and static stretching are well-tolerated forms of therapy for people with tennis elbow.

The Two Exercises That Can Help Repair Your Damaged Tendon

The first exercise I'm going to go over is the *static* stretch that was used in so many of the studies we've just gone over. A static (or stationary) stretch takes the muscle and tendon, puts it in a lengthened position, and keeps it there for a certain period of time. It goes like this:

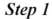

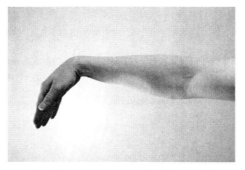

- hold your arm out in front of you
- make sure your elbow is straight

Step2

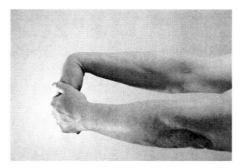

- with your other hand, *gently* pull your wrist *slowly* into a bent position
- stop when you feel a gentle stretch
- mild pain is okay, but no more than that
- hold for 30 seconds, then slowly release

The second exercise is the *eccentric weight training exercise*, also used in the previously mentioned studies. There's a few more details to cover about this exercise than the static stretch, so I'll present this information in a question and answer format–simply because it's just plain easier to digest that way. So, first off…

What kind of weight will I need?

Since it's a *weight* training exercise, it's a no brainer that you're going to need a weight to use. In my experience treating patients, the easiest thing to do is to just go to a sporting goods store (or large retail store), and purchase several light dumbbells. Most look something like this:

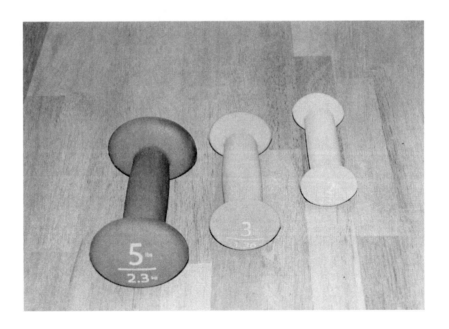

Light dumbbells such as these are inexpensive, which is a good thing, because you're going to need to get several different sizes as you progress with the exercise program. Of course you technically can use any kind of weight that's comfortable to grip and allows you to progress to a heavier weight in small increments.

How much weight should I start off with?

How much weight you start out using on the eccentric exercise will depend on how much pain you're having *and* how strong you are. If you were sitting in my treatment booth, I would have to test you with several dumbbells to figure out what weight is right for you to begin with.

My trial and error process would go something like this. I'd first have you move your wrist up and down to see how painful this motion is for you to do. If you were hurting a lot when doing this motion with *no weight*, then obviously you would start out with no weight.

On the other hand, if you could move your wrist up and down okay, and it didn't bother you that much, I'd hand you a one-pound dumbbell and have you try that. If the one-pound dumbbell felt fine and seemed too light, we'd simply keep repeating this process until we found a size dumbbell that a) wasn't too light, and b) caused no more than mild pain when moving your wrist up and down. At this point, we now have a reasonable starting place, and I'd next have you actually try the eccentric exercise with that particular dumbbell to make sure that we've got the right weight for you. If not, we'd just "tweak" things as necessary by going up or down a pound or so.

My suggestion is to try this trial and error process briefly in the store when choosing a dumbbell if at all possible. It takes just a few minutes to grip a dumbbell, move your wrist up and down, and try out a few different sizes. If you get home and find out that you really need a lighter or heavier weight, most stores will let you gladly exchange them–so save that receipt!

How many times will I have to lower the dumbbell?

In order to answer this question, I probably need to go over several weight-training terms first–just to make sure that no one will get lost as we're covering the guidelines. The two in particular you need to be familiar with are *repetition* and *set*.

First, what is a repetition? Well, when it comes to eccentric training, if you take a weight and lower it, you could say that you have just done one repetition or "rep" of that exercise. Likewise, if you take the same weight and lower it a total of ten times, then you could say that you did ten repetitions of that exercise.

A set, on the other hand, is simply a bunch of repetitions done one after the other. Using our above example once again, if you lowered a weight ten times in a row, and then rested, you would have just done one set of ten repetitions.

Okay, so now that we're all on the same page, every reader will now understand my answer to the question, "How many times will I have to lower the dumbbell?" And the answer is that you need to do three sets of ten repetitions of each exercise, which we could write as 3 sets x 10 reps.

Note that if you cannot do three full sets of ten, simply work up to it. For example, if you can only do three sets of *six* repetitions, next time see if you can do three sets of eight or nine repetitions. Likewise, if you can do only *two* sets of ten repetitions, work up to doing the third set. Whatever the case, work up to the three sets of ten if you have to.

Now some readers may be wondering where I got these numbers from. Well, they're taken right from the published research studies we've just been going over. Since the majority of the controlled trials on tennis elbow and eccentric training have had subjects do three sets of ten reps, those are the numbers we're going with. As the saying goes, if it ain't broke, don't fix it…

How much pain should I be in when doing the exercises?

Something you definitely need to know about as some might be inclined to use the "no-pain, no gain" philosophy when doing the exercises. Well, that's not the thing to do when rehabilitating tennis elbow.

Perhaps the best way to tell you how much discomfort is okay to have when doing the exercises is to put it like this: continue to exercise even if you experience *mild* pain, but **stop** an exercise if the pain becomes disabling. In other words, a little pain or discomfort is acceptable, but that's about it. This is the guideline used in studies that have had no dropouts so it's a good rule of thumb to go by.

Okay. Now that you know some of the basic guidelines for the eccentric exercise, here's how it's done...

Step 1

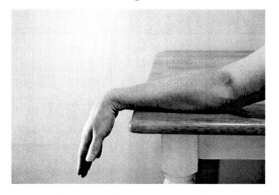

- sit in a chair next to a table that allows you to put your arm in the above position

Step2

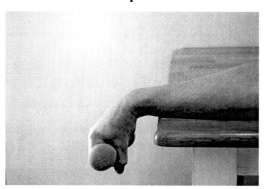

- place the dumbbell in your hand with your good arm

Step 3

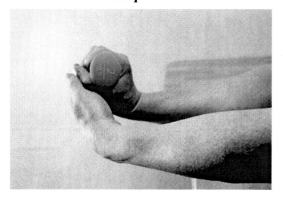

- lift the dumbbell up as high as you can comfortably with your good hand
- the hand with the dumbbell in it tries not to help out at all with this raising motion

Step 4

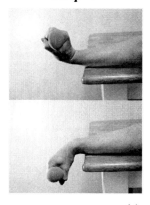

- now remove your good hand and let the hand with the dumbbell lower the weight down slowly as far as is comfortable
- you've just done one repetition
- now go back to Step 3 and repeat for a total of 10 times in a row
- after you've done a set of ten repetitions, rest about 1 minute
- do 2 more sets with about 1 minute of rest between sets for a total of 3 sets

The Routine

Now that you're familiar with all the exercises, it's time to put them together into one routine. When all is said and done, here's what it looks like…

**Do the following routine on *MONDAY, WEDNESDAY, and FRIDAY*
<u>or</u> *TUESDAY, THURSDAY and SATURDAY***

Static Stretch	**Eccentric Exercise**	**Static Stretch**

-hold for 30 seconds
-rest for 30 seconds
-repeat for a total of 3 times
	-work up to doing
	  3 sets x 10 repetitons
	-rest 1minute between
	  sets
		-hold for 30 seconds
		-rest for 30 seconds
		-repeat for a total of 3 times

Track Your Progress!

Since it can be hard to remember from one session to the next what weight you used and how many reps you did for each set, it's helpful to quickly jot down this information. The following is an example of how to keep track of your progress by using the exercise sheets provided at the end of this section.

start with three 30-second static stretches

#1 ✓   rest 30 seconds   #2 ✓   rest 30 seconds   #3 ✓

Eccentric Exercise: work up to 3 sets x 10 reps

	weight used	number of repetitions you did
Set #1	2 lb.	10
Set #2	2 lb.	10
Set #3	2 lb.	8

end with three 30-second static stretches

#1 ✓   rest 30 seconds   #2 ✓   rest 30 seconds   #3 ✓

As you can see, this person is using a two pound dumbbell and was able to do two sets of ten repetitions, but on the third set, was only able to do eight. This means that next session they should try to progress to doing nine or ten repetitions on the third set *if* their symptoms allow. And once they can do three sets of ten repetitions without much discomfort, it is time to switch to a one or two pound *heavier* dumbbell.

The pages that follow contain exercise sheets for eight-weeks of workouts. Make additional copies as needed. A **Quickstart Guide** is included on page 62 at the end of this chapter to get you started.

Week 1: Exercise Session #1

start with three 30-second static stretches

#1_____   rest 30 seconds   #2_____   rest 30 seconds   #3 _____

Eccentric Exercise: work up to 3 sets x 10 reps

	weight used	number of repetitions you did
Set #1	_____	_____
Set #2	_____	_____
Set #3	_____	_____

end with three 30-second static stretches

#1_____   rest 30 seconds   #2_____   rest 30 seconds   #3 _____

Week 1: Exercise Session #2

start with three 30-second static stretches

#1_____   rest 30 seconds   #2_____   rest 30 seconds   #3 _____

Eccentric Exercise: work up to 3 sets x 10 reps

	weight used	number of repetitions you did
Set #1	_____	_____
Set #2	_____	_____
Set #3	_____	_____

end with three 30-second static stretches

#1_____   rest 30 seconds   #2_____   rest 30 seconds   #3 _____

Week 1: Exercise Session #3

start with three 30-second static stretches

#1_____   rest 30 seconds   #2_____   rest 30 seconds   #3 _____

Eccentric Exercise: work up to 3 sets x 10 reps

	weight used	number of repetitions you did
Set #1	_____	_____
Set #2	_____	_____
Set #3	_____	_____

end with three 30-second static stretches

#1_____   rest 30 seconds   #2_____   rest 30 seconds   #3 _____

Week 2: Exercise Session #1

start with three 30-second static stretches

#1_____   rest 30 seconds   #2_____   rest 30 seconds   #3 _____

Eccentric Exercise: work up to 3 sets x 10 reps

	weight used	number of repetitions you did
Set #1	_____	_____
Set #2	_____	_____
Set #3	_____	_____

end with three 30-second static stretches

#1_____   rest 30 seconds   #2_____   rest 30 seconds   #3 _____

Week 2: Exercise Session #2

start with three 30-second static stretches

#1_____   rest 30 seconds   #2_____   rest 30 seconds   #3 _____

Eccentric Exercise: work up to 3 sets x 10 reps

	weight used	number of repetitions you did
Set #1	_____	_____
Set #2	_____	_____
Set #3	_____	_____

end with three 30-second static stretches

#1_____   rest 30 seconds   #2_____   rest 30 seconds   #3 _____

Week 2: Exercise Session #3

start with three 30-second static stretches

#1_____   rest 30 seconds   #2_____   rest 30 seconds   #3 _____

Eccentric Exercise: work up to 3 sets x 10 reps

	weight used	number of repetitions you did
Set #1	_____	_____
Set #2	_____	_____
Set #3	_____	_____

end with three 30-second static stretches

#1_____   rest 30 seconds   #2_____   rest 30 seconds   #3 _____

Week 3: Exercise Session #1

start with three 30-second static stretches

#1_____   rest 30 seconds   #2_____   rest 30 seconds   #3 _____

Eccentric Exercise: work up to 3 sets x 10 reps

	weight used	number of repetitions you did
Set #1	_____	_____
Set #2	_____	_____
Set #3	_____	_____

end with three 30-second static stretches

#1_____   rest 30 seconds   #2_____   rest 30 seconds   #3 _____

Week 3: Exercise Session #2

start with three 30-second static stretches

#1_____   rest 30 seconds   #2_____   rest 30 seconds   #3 _____

Eccentric Exercise: work up to 3 sets x 10 reps

	weight used	number of repetitions you did
Set #1	_____	_____
Set #2	_____	_____
Set #3	_____	_____

end with three 30-second static stretches

#1_____   rest 30 seconds   #2_____   rest 30 seconds   #3 _____

Week 3: Exercise Session #3

<u>start with three 30-second static stretches</u>

#1_____   rest 30 seconds   #2_____   rest 30 seconds   #3 _____

<u>Eccentric Exercise: work up to 3 sets x 10 reps</u>

weight used   number of repetitions you did

Set #1   _____   _____

Set #2   _____   _____

Set #3   _____   _____

<u>end with three 30-second static stretches</u>

#1_____   rest 30 seconds   #2_____   rest 30 seconds   #3 _____

Week 4: Exercise Session #1

<u>start with three 30-second static stretches</u>

#1_____   rest 30 seconds   #2_____   rest 30 seconds   #3 _____

<u>Eccentric Exercise: work up to 3 sets x 10 reps</u>

weight used   number of repetitions you did

Set #1   _____   _____

Set #2   _____   _____

Set #3   _____   _____

<u>end with three 30-second static stretches</u>

#1_____   rest 30 seconds   #2_____   rest 30 seconds   #3 _____

Week 4: Exercise Session #2

start with three 30-second static stretches

#1_____   rest 30 seconds   #2_____   rest 30 seconds   #3 _____

Eccentric Exercise: work up to 3 sets x 10 reps

	weight used	number of repetitions you did
Set #1	_____	_____
Set #2	_____	_____
Set #3	_____	_____

end with three 30-second static stretches

#1_____   rest 30 seconds   #2_____   rest 30 seconds   #3 _____

Week 4: Exercise Session #3

start with three 30-second static stretches

#1_____   rest 30 seconds   #2_____   rest 30 seconds   #3 _____

Eccentric Exercise: work up to 3 sets x 10 reps

	weight used	number of repetitions you did
Set #1	_____	_____
Set #2	_____	_____
Set #3	_____	_____

end with three 30-second static stretches

#1_____   rest 30 seconds   #2_____   rest 30 seconds   #3 _____

Week 5: Exercise Session #1

<u>start with three 30-second static stretches</u>

#1_____   rest 30 seconds   #2_____   rest 30 seconds   #3 _____

<u>Eccentric Exercise: work up to 3 sets x 10 reps</u>

	weight used	number of repetitions you did
Set #1	_____	_____
Set #2	_____	_____
Set #3	_____	_____

<u>end with three 30-second static stretches</u>

#1_____   rest 30 seconds   #2_____   rest 30 seconds   #3 _____

Week 5: Exercise Session #2

<u>start with three 30-second static stretches</u>

#1_____   rest 30 seconds   #2_____   rest 30 seconds   #3 _____

<u>Eccentric Exercise: work up to 3 sets x 10 reps</u>

	weight used	number of repetitions you did
Set #1	_____	_____
Set #2	_____	_____
Set #3	_____	_____

<u>end with three 30-second static stretches</u>

#1_____   rest 30 seconds   #2_____   rest 30 seconds   #3 _____

Week 5: Exercise Session #3

start with three 30-second static stretches

#1_____   rest 30 seconds   #2_____   rest 30 seconds   #3 _____

Eccentric Exercise: work up to 3 sets x 10 reps

	weight used	number of repetitions you did
Set #1	_____	_____
Set #2	_____	_____
Set #3	_____	_____

end with three 30-second static stretches

#1_____   rest 30 seconds   #2_____   rest 30 seconds   #3 _____

Week 6: Exercise Session #1

start with three 30-second static stretches

#1_____   rest 30 seconds   #2_____   rest 30 seconds   #3 _____

Eccentric Exercise: work up to 3 sets x 10 reps

	weight used	number of repetitions you did
Set #1	_____	_____
Set #2	_____	_____
Set #3	_____	_____

end with three 30-second static stretches

#1_____   rest 30 seconds   #2_____   rest 30 seconds   #3 _____

Week 6: Exercise Session #2

start with three 30-second static stretches

#1_____   rest 30 seconds   #2_____   rest 30 seconds   #3 _____

Eccentric Exercise: work up to 3 sets x 10 reps

	weight used	number of repetitions you did
Set #1	_____	_____
Set #2	_____	_____
Set #3	_____	_____

end with three 30-second static stretches

#1_____   rest 30 seconds   #2_____   rest 30 seconds   #3 _____

Week 6: Exercise Session #3

start with three 30-second static stretches

#1_____   rest 30 seconds   #2_____   rest 30 seconds   #3 _____

Eccentric Exercise: work up to 3 sets x 10 reps

	weight used	number of repetitions you did
Set #1	_____	_____
Set #2	_____	_____
Set #3	_____	_____

end with three 30-second static stretches

#1_____   rest 30 seconds   #2_____   rest 30 seconds   #3 _____

Week 7: Exercise Session #1

start with three 30-second static stretches

#1_____   rest 30 seconds   #2_____   rest 30 seconds   #3 _____

Eccentric Exercise: work up to 3 sets x 10 reps

	weight used	number of repetitions you did
Set #1	_____	_____
Set #2	_____	_____
Set #3	_____	_____

end with three 30-second static stretches

#1_____   rest 30 seconds   #2_____   rest 30 seconds   #3 _____

Week 7: Exercise Session #2

start with three 30-second static stretches

#1_____   rest 30 seconds   #2_____   rest 30 seconds   #3 _____

Eccentric Exercise: work up to 3 sets x 10 reps

	weight used	number of repetitions you did
Set #1	_____	_____
Set #2	_____	_____
Set #3	_____	_____

end with three 30-second static stretches

#1_____   rest 30 seconds   #2_____   rest 30 seconds   #3 _____

Week 7: Exercise Session #3

start with three 30-second static stretches

#1_____   rest 30 seconds   #2_____   rest 30 seconds   #3 _____

Eccentric Exercise: work up to 3 sets x 10 reps

	weight used	number of repetitions you did
Set #1	_____	_____
Set #2	_____	_____
Set #3	_____	_____

end with three 30-second static stretches

#1_____   rest 30 seconds   #2_____   rest 30 seconds   #3 _____

Week 8: Exercise Session #1

start with three 30-second static stretches

#1_____   rest 30 seconds   #2_____   rest 30 seconds   #3 _____

Eccentric Exercise: work up to 3 sets x 10 reps

	weight used	number of repetitions you did
Set #1	_____	_____
Set #2	_____	_____
Set #3	_____	_____

end with three 30-second static stretches

#1_____   rest 30 seconds   #2_____   rest 30 seconds   #3 _____

Week 8: Exercise Session #2

start with three 30-second static stretches

#1_____   rest 30 seconds   #2_____   rest 30 seconds   #3 _____

Eccentric Exercise: work up to 3 sets x 10 reps

	weight used	number of repetitions you did
Set #1	_____	_____
Set #2	_____	_____
Set #3	_____	_____

end with three 30-second static stretches

#1_____   rest 30 seconds   #2_____   rest 30 seconds   #3 _____

Week 8: Exercise Session #3

start with three 30-second static stretches

#1_____   rest 30 seconds   #2_____   rest 30 seconds   #3 _____

Eccentric Exercise: work up to 3 sets x 10 reps

	weight used	number of repetitions you did
Set #1	_____	_____
Set #2	_____	_____
Set #3	_____	_____

end with three 30-second static stretches

#1_____   rest 30 seconds   #2_____   rest 30 seconds   #3 _____

Quickstart Guide

- ✓ purchase several light dumbbells

- ✓ use the trial and error process described on page 45 to choose the correct weight to start off with

- ✓ familiarize yourself with the exercises by reviewing the steps on pages 43 and 47

- ✓ begin exercising

- ✓ it is okay to start off doing the eccentric exercise with no weight if you have to

- ✓ it is also okay to wear the counterforce brace while doing the eccentric exercise. However try exercising without it now and then, and stop using it when you are able to.

- ✓ it is okay to have *mild* pain while exercising but stop if the pain becomes disabling

- ✓ chart your progress using the handy exercise sheets provided

- ✓ when you can do three sets of ten repetitions without much discomfort, it is time to switch to a one or two pound heavier dumbbell

- ✓ try to stick with the routine for at least 4 to 8 weeks for best results

Measure Your Progress

Okay. You've learned all about tennis elbow, have started using one or both of the strategies described in Chapters 4 and 5, and are on the road to recovery. So now what should you expect?

Well, we all know you should expect to get better. But what exactly does *better* mean? As a physical therapist treating patients, it means two distinct things to me:

- your arm starts to *feel* better

and

- your arm starts to *work* better

And so, when a patient returns for a follow-up visit, I re-assess them, looking for specific changes in their arm pain, as well as their arm function.

In this book, I'm going to recommend that readers do the same thing periodically. Why? Simply because people in pain can't always see the progress they're making. For instance sometimes a person's pain is exactly the same, but they aren't aware that they can now actually do some motions or tasks that they couldn't do before–a sure sign that things are healing. *Or*, sometimes a person still has significant pain but they're not aware that it's actually occurring less frequently–yet another good indication that positive changes are taking place.

Whatever the case may be, if a person isn't looking at the bigger picture, and doesn't *think* they're getting any better, they're likely to get discouraged and stop doing the exercises altogether–even though they really might have been on the right track!

On the other hand though, what if you periodically check your progress and are keenly aware that your arm has made some changes for the better? What if you can *positively* see objective results? My guess is that you're going to be giving yourself a healthy dose of motivation to keep on stickin' with the program.

Having said that, I'm going to show you exactly what to check for from time to time so that you can monitor *all* the changes that are taking place in your arm. I call them "outcomes" and there are two of them.

Outcome #1:
Look for Changes in Your Pain

First of all, you should look for changes in your pain. I know this may sound silly, but sometimes it's my job to get a person to see that their pain *is* actually improving. You see, a lot of people come to physical therapy thinking they're going to be pain-free right away. Then, when they're not instantly better and still having pain, they often start to worry and become discouraged. Truth is, I have seen very few people start an exercise program and get instantly better. Better yes, but not *instantly* better.

Over the years, I have found that patients usually respond to therapy in a quite predictable pattern. One of three things will almost always occur as a person begins to turn the corner and get better:

- your arm pain is just as intense as always, however now it is occurring much less frequently

  or

- your arm pain is now *less* intense, even though it still occurring just as frequently

  or

- you start to notice less intense arm pain *and* it is now occurring less frequently

The point here is to make sure that you keep a sharp eye out for these three scenarios as you continue with the exercises. If *any* of them occur, it will be a sure sign that the program is working. You can then look forward to the pain gradually getting better, usually over the weeks to come.

Outcome #2:
Look for Changes in Arm Function

Looking at how well your arm works is very important because sometimes arm function improves *before* the pain does. For example, sometimes a patient will do the exercises for a while, and although their arm will still hurt a lot, they are able to do many activities that they haven't been able to in a while–a really good indicator that healing is taking place *and* that the pain should be easing up soon.

While measuring your arm function may sound like a pain in the butt, it doesn't have to be. In this book, I'm recommending that readers use a quick and easy assessment tool known as *The Patient-Rated Tennis Elbow Evaluation,* or for short, the PRTEE.

Developed by Joy MacDermid, the PRTEE has actually been around for awhile and was specially made to document pain and disability in tennis elbow patients. It is very well researched and has been shown to be:

- *valid*, meaning that it actually measures what it's supposed to be measuring (Newcomer 2005)

- *reliable*, meaning that you can get the same result with repeated testing (Overend 1999)

- *responsive*, meaning that it has the ability to detect changes in a person over time (Newcomer 2005)

Additionally, the PRTEE takes about 5 minutes to complete and can be scored with a simple calculator in under a minute. Now that's my kinda test!

So what exactly does the PRTEE involve? Not much. You simply go down a list of 15 items, circling the number to the right that best applies to your particular situation. Then, when you've done that, you simply perform a few easy calculations to see how many points you have out of a possible 100.

And what do the numbers mean? Well, this is one of the few times in your life where getting a hundred is not good. While 100 is the highest number you can score on the PRTEE, it's also *the worst* you can possibly do. This means you are having *much* pain and disability.

Likewise, a zero is the lowest score and means you are having no pain or disability. On the next page is a copy of the PRTEE.

THE PATIENT-RATED TENNIS ELBOW EVALUATION
(or the PRTEE for short)

*The questions below will help us understand the amount of difficulty you have had with your arm in the past week. You will be describing your **average** arm symptoms **over the past week** on a scale 0-10. Please provide an answer for all questions. If you did not perform an activity because of pain or because you were unable then you should circle a "10". If you are unsure please estimate to the best of your ability. Only leave items blank if you never perform that activity. Please indicate this by drawing a line completely through the question.*

1. PAIN in your affected arm

*Rate the average amount of pain in your arm **over the past week** by circling the number that best describes your pain on a scale from 0-10. A **zero (0)** means that you **did not have any pain** and a **ten (10)** means that you had **the worst pain imaginable.***

RATE YOUR PAIN: No Pain	Worst Imaginable
When your are at rest	0　1　2　3　4　5　6　7　8　9　10
When doing a task with repeated arm movement	0　1　2　3　4　5　6　7　8　9　10
When carrying a plastic bag of groceries	0　1　2　3　4　5　6　7　8　9　10
When your pain was at its least	0　1　2　3　4　5　6　7　8　9　10
When your pain was at its worst	0　1　2　3　4　5　6　7　8　9　10

Now, add up the circled numbers to get Total #1_____

2. FUNCTIONAL DISABILITY		

A. SPECIFIC ACTIVITIES

    *Rate the **amount of difficulty** you experienced performing each of the tasks listed below, over the past week, by circling the number that best describes your difficulty on a scale of 0-10. A <u>zero (0)</u> means you <u>did not experience any difficulty</u> and a **ten (10)** means it was **so difficult you were unable to do it at all**.*

	No Difficulty Unable To Do
Turn a doorknob or key	0 1 2 3 4 5 6 7 8 9 10
Carry a grocery bag or briefcase by the handle	0 1 2 3 4 5 6 7 8 9 10
Lift a full coffee cup or glass of milk to your mouth	0 1 2 3 4 5 6 7 8 9 10
Open a jar	0 1 2 3 4 5 6 7 8 9 10
Pull up pants	0 1 2 3 4 5 6 7 8 9 10
Wring out a washcloth or wet towel	0 1 2 3 4 5 6 7 8 9 10

B. USUAL ACTIVITIES

    *Rate the **amount of difficulty** you experienced performing your **usual** activities in each of the areas listed below, over the past week, by circling the number that best describes your difficulty on a scale of 0-10. By "usual activities", we mean the activities that you performed **before** you started having a problem with your arm. A **zero** (0) means you did not experience any difficulty and a **ten** (10) means it was so difficult you were unable to do any of your usual activities.*

1. Personal activities (dressing, washing)	0 1 2 3 4 5 6 7 8 9 10
2. Household work (cleaning, maintenance)	0 1 2 3 4 5 6 7 8 9 10
3. Work (your job or everyday work)	0 1 2 3 4 5 6 7 8 9 10
4. Recreational or sporting activities	0 1 2 3 4 5 6 7 8 9 10

Now, add up the circled numbers, and then divide by 2 to get Total #2_____

Last step: add up Total #1 and Total #2 to get your Score_____

So how'd you do? Remember, the lower the number, the better your pain and function–which is what you want to shoot for. If you scored in the single digits, such as 3 or 5, you probably don't need this book too much.

On the other hand, higher scores, such as 85 or 95, show us that your tennis elbow is pretty bad. And if you did score this high, don't worry. Just re-take the PRTEE every few weeks or so, and as you continue with the exercises, you should see your score go lower and lower as time passes. Remember, often times arm function gets better *before* the pain does.

Key Points

✓ being aware of your progress is an important part of treating your own tennis elbow–it motivates you to keep doing the exercises

✓ look for the pain to become less *intense*, less *frequent*, or both to let you know that the exercises are helping

✓ sometimes your arm starts to work better *before* it starts to feel better. Taking the PRTEE from time to time makes you aware of these improvements.

Comprehensive List of Supporting References

It's true! All the information in this book is based on randomized controlled trials and scientific studies that have been published in peer-reviewed journals. Since I know there are readers out there that like to actually check out the information for themselves, I've included the references for every study I have cited in this book...

Chapter 1

De Zordo T, et al. Real-time sonoelastography of lateral epicondylitis: comparison of findings between patients and healthy volunteers. *American Journal of Roentgenology* 2009;193:180-5.

McFarland G B, et al. Kinesiology of selected muscles acting on the wrist: electromyographic study. *Archives of Physical Medicine and Rehabilitation* 1962;43:165-171.

Morris H. Lawn-tennis elbow. *The British Medical Journal* 1883;2(1185): 557.

Nirschl R, et al. Tennis elbow. The surgical treatment of lateral epicondylitis. *The Journal of Bone and Joint Surgery* 1979;61-A:832-839.

Potter H, et al. Lateral epicondylitis; correlation of MR imaging, surgical, and histopathologic findings. *Radiology* 1995;196:43-6.

Radonjic D, et al. Kinesiology of the wrist. *American Journal of Physical Medicine* 1971;50:57-71.

Regan W, et al. Microscopic histopathology of chronic refractory lateral epicondylitis. *The American Journal of Sports Medicine* 1992;20:746-749.

Chapter 2

Nirschl R, et al. Tennis elbow. The surgical treatment of lateral epicondylitis. *The Journal of Bone and Joint Surgery* 1979;61-A:832-839.

Potter H, et al. Lateral epicondylitis; correlation of MR imaging, surgical, and histopathologic findings. *Radiology* 1995;196:43-6.

Regan W, et al. Microscopic histopathology of chronic refractory lateral epicondylitis. *The American Journal of Sports Medicine* 1992;20:746-749.

Verhaar J, et al. Lateral extensor release for tennis elbow. A prospective long-term follow-up study. *Journal of Bone and Joint Surgery* 1993;75-A:1034-43.

Chapter 3

Bisset L, et al. Mobilisation with movement and exercise, corticosteroid injection, or wait and see for tennis elbow: randomised trial. *British Medical Journal* 2006;333:939-945.

Smidt N, et al. Corticosteroid injections, physiotherapy, or a wait-and-see policy for lateral epicondylitis: a randomised controlled trial. *The Lancet* 2002;359:657-662.

Chapter 4

Burton, AK. Grip strength and forearm straps in tennis elbow. *British Journal of Sports Medicine* 1985;19:37-38.

Haker E, et al. Elbow-band, splintage and steroids in lateral epicondylalgia (tennis elbow). *The Pain Clinic* 1993;6:103-112.

Ng, GYF, et al. The immediate effects of tension of counterforce forearm brace on neuromuscular performance of wrist extensor muscles in subjects with lateral humeral epicondylosis. *Journal of Orthopaedic and Sports Physical Therapy* 2004;34:72-78.

Struijs P, et al. Conservative treatment of lateral epicondylitis. Brace versus physical therapy or a combination of both-a randomized clinical trial. *The American Journal of Sports Medicine* 2004;32:462-469.

Wadsworth CT, et al. Effect of the counterforce armband on wrist extension and grip strength and pain in subjects with tennis elbow. *Journal of Orthopaedic and Sports Physical Therapy* 1989;11:192-197.

Chapter 5

Manias P, et al. A controlled clinical pilot trial to study the effectiveness of ice as a supplement to the exercise programme for the management of lateral elbow tendinopathy. *British Journal of Sports Medicine* 2006;40:81-85.

Martinez-Silvestrini J, et al. Chronic lateral epicondylitis: comparative effectiveness of a home exercise program including stretching alone versus stretching supplemented with eccentric or concentric strengthening. *Journal of Hand Therapy* 2005;18:411-419.

Pienimaki T, et al. Progressive strengthening and stretching exercises and ultrasound for chronic lateral epicondylitis. *Physiotherapy* 1996;82;522-530.

Stasinopoulos D, et al. Comparison of effects of Cyriax physiotherapy, a supervised exercise programme and polarized polychromatic non-coherent light (Bioptron light) for the treatment of lateral epicondylitis. *Clinical Rehabilitation* 2006;20:12-23.

Chapter 6

Newcomer, K, et al. Sensitivity of the patient-rated forearm evaluation questionnaire in lateral epicondylitis. *Journal of Hand Therapy* 2005;18:400-406.

Overend T, et al. Reliability of a patient-rated forearm evaluation questionnaire for patients with lateral epicondylitis. *Journal of Hand Therapy* 1999;12:31-37.

CPSIA information can be obtained at www.ICGtesting.com
Printed in the USA
268942BV00005B/6/P